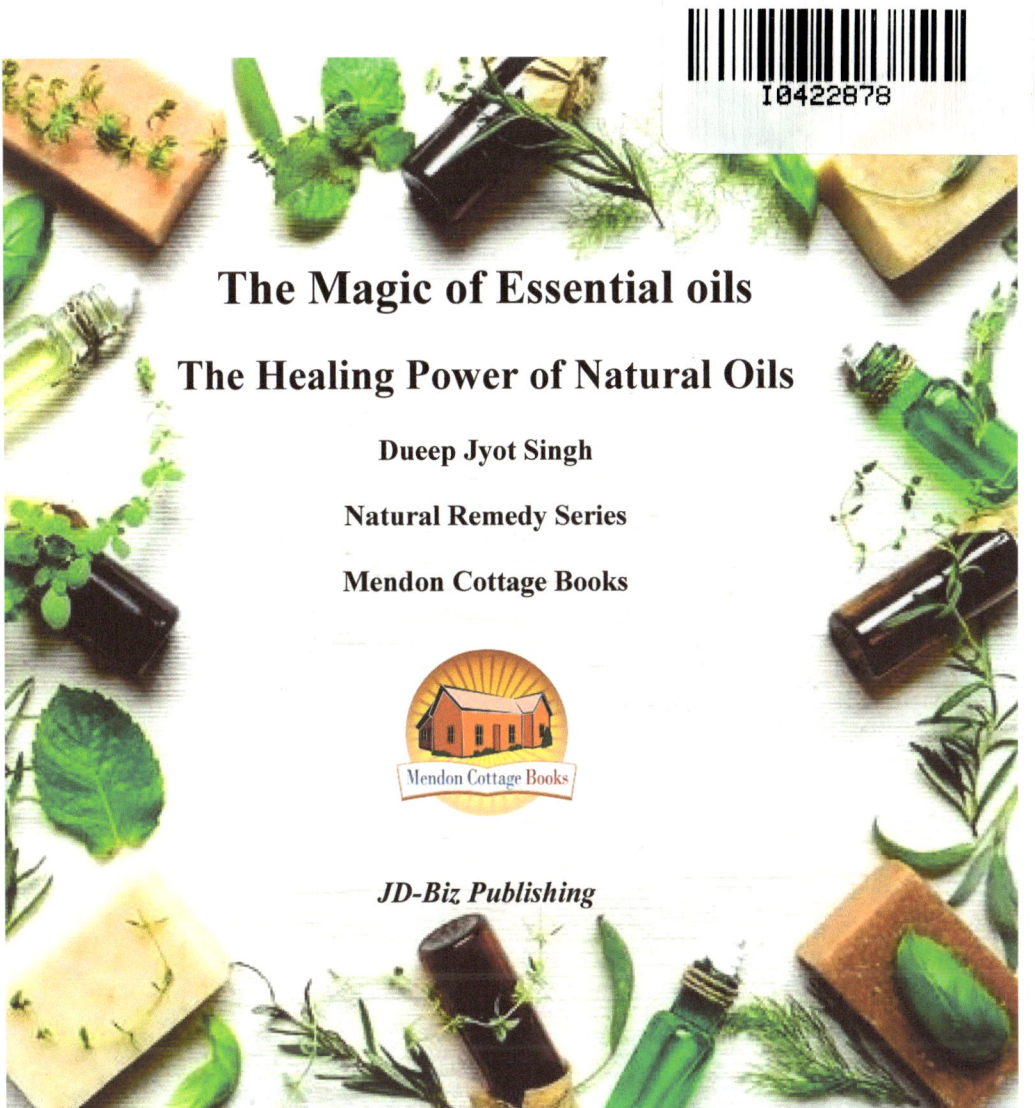

# The Magic of Essential oils

## The Healing Power of Natural Oils

**Dueep Jyot Singh**

**Natural Remedy Series**

**Mendon Cottage Books**

Mendon Cottage Books

*JD-Biz Publishing*

**Disclaimer**

The information is this book is provided for informational purposes only. It is not intended to be used and medical advice or a substitute for proper medical treatment by a qualified health care provider. The information is believed to be accurate as presented based on research by the author.

The contents have not been evaluated by the U.S. Food and Drug Administration or any other Government or Health Organization and the contents in this book are not to be used to treat cure or prevent disease.

The author or publisher is not responsible for the use or safety of any diet, procedure or treatment mentioned in this book. The author or publisher is not responsible for errors or omissions that may exist.

**Warning**

The Book is for informational purposes only and before taking on any diet, treatment or medical procedure, it is recommended to consult with your primary health care provider.

Our books are available at

1. Amazon.com

2. Barnes and Noble

3. Itunes

4. Kobo

5. Smashwords

6. Google Play Books

# Table of Contents

# Introduction

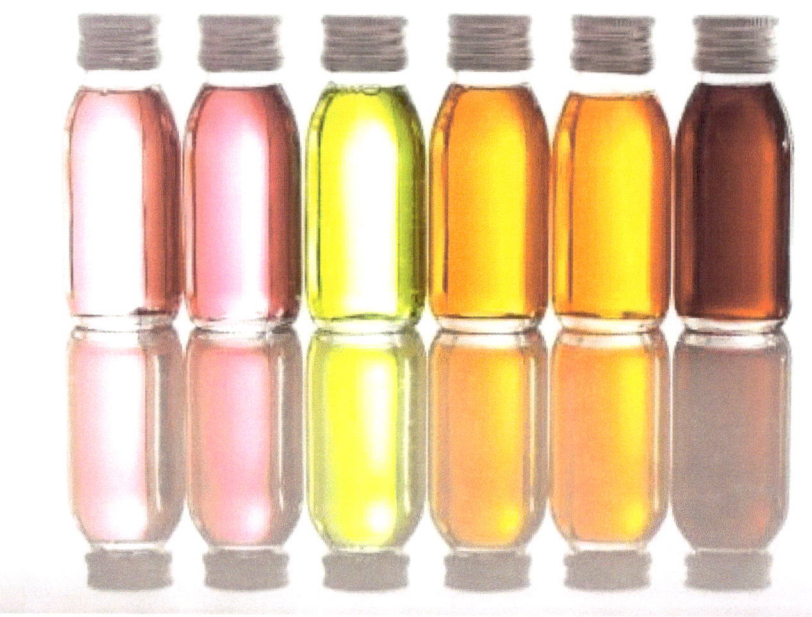

Eastern history, going back to the 14 – 16 century talks about how Rose oil was "discovered" by the future Empress Noorjahan when she was living in the harem of the Mogul Emperor Jahangir. It seems she saw essential oils floating on the surface of the water pools where rose petals floated day in day out. She asked some slaves to collect that oily liquid and began to make perfumes for the other ladies of the harem. And so the essential oil and perfume industry was born in the Indian subcontinent.

Sherlock Holmes is going to raise an eyebrow at this story. "My dear Watson, this story is a figment of the Eastern imagination. Unless of course we supposed the rooms to be so boiling hot that the steeped petals released their essential oils. Or the room temperature of those closed up areas was so high that steam condensed to get Rosewater and Rose oil. And one knows that the art of distilling and extracting essential oils has been known to the wise men and women of the East and of the best for millenniums. They have been using these essential oils for aromatherapy, for massage oils, for tinctures, lotions, ointments, decoctions and any other beauty or herbal remedies. So I will take this Rose oil, and the Empress story with a pinch of salt. QED. Where is my violin?"

Since ancient times, human beings understood that plants had something in them, which could be used, through extraction. This magic product was oils. There are two types of essential oils obtained from plants – volatile oils and fixed oils.

# Difference between Volatile Oils and Fixed Oils

The oils that you call essential oils are volatile oils. Fixed oils are found in the seeds, and in the nuts, and are obtained by pressing. The essential oils are the aromatic fragrances obtained through treating leaves, bark, flowers, and the roots of the plant. These oils are normally present in the oil glands of the plant tissue.

Volatile oils are definitely more difficult to obtain, because they need to be distilled over a solvent. That is the reason why, these volatile essential oils are so expensive. They are also as the name says, volatile, and do not keep for long periods of time, unless preserved with other preserving oil mixtures.

On the other hand, fixed oils, which are natural oils, which are obtained through oil pressing, last long, really long. These are the oils, which you use for making beautifying lotions, potions, ointments, and for other purposes, including healing salves.

The cost of essential oils definitely vary upon the process used to extract that particular oil, and the quality of oil obtained. Good quality essential oils, especially flower extracts are extremely expensive, because around 60,000 roses are going to go in the extraction of 1 g of Rose essential oil.

Essential oils are extremely strong, because they are so powerful and concentrated. That is why it is necessary to dilute them, before you use them. However, the diluting process can be done extremely easily by infusing the oils from all these aromatic plants. These infused oils do not need to be diluted, because the essential oil has already been suffused in the infusion.

Besides this, infused oils do not concentrate on just one part of the plant – that being its essential oil. It takes the beneficial value of the complete plant as a whole.

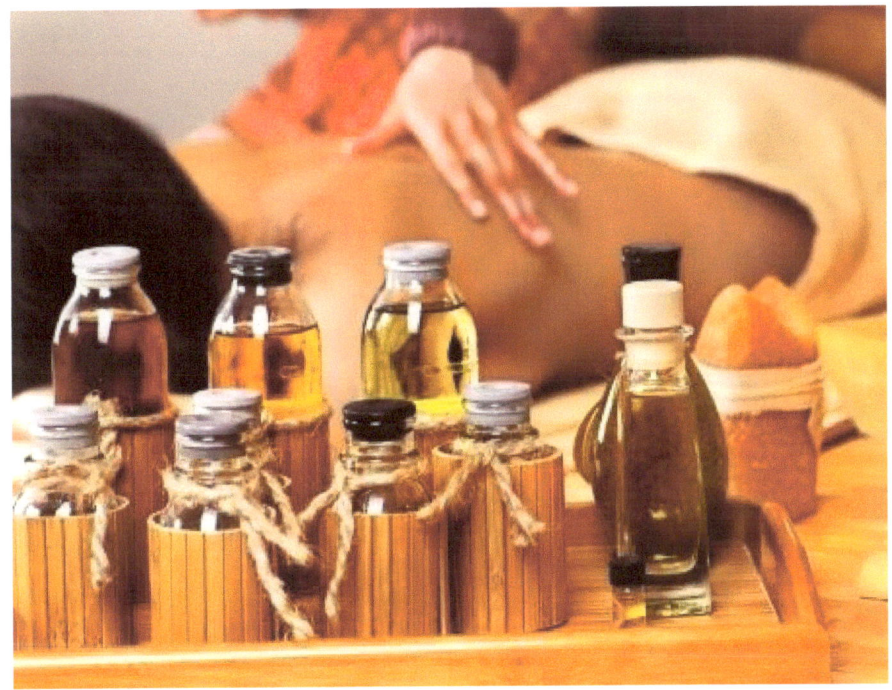

**Essential Oils have been in use since ancient times to keep one healthy and beautiful**

The best fixed oils are the ones which are obtained through cold pressing. However, nowadays, many of these oils are subjected to different procedures of extraction, including emulsification, solidification, and heating. This removes plenty of the natural qualities of the fixed oils, and also retracts from their beneficial healthy qualities.

Fixed oils are going to oxidize over the passage of time and that is why you can prevent them from becoming rancid by adding 5 to 10% of wheat germ oil. You can also add 5% of vitamin E oil, especially if you are using that particular fixed oil to make a skin beautifying ointment.

# Essential Oils in Aromatherapy

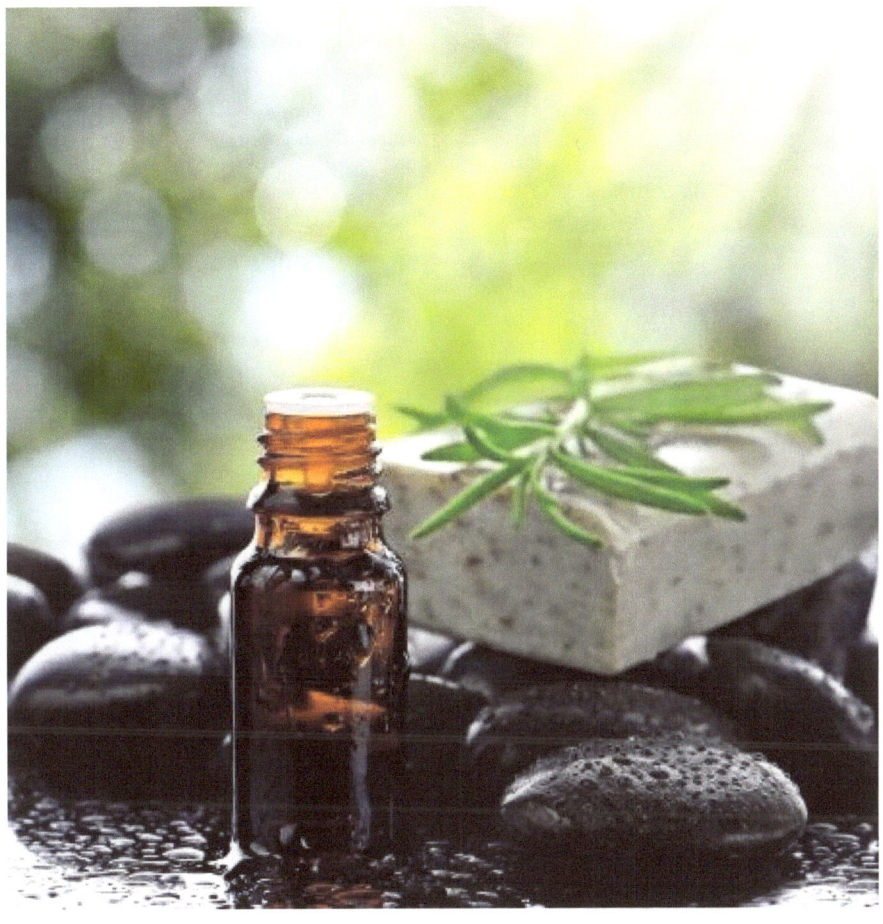

When you talk about essential oils, can aroma therapy be far behind? The term aromatherapy was used for the first time in 1937 by a chemist in his book *Aromathérapie: Les Huiles Essentielles, Hormones Végétales* written by René-Maurice Gattefossé. But before that, this amazingly effective alternative medicine form was in use in the East and in the West, to heal and cure people, mentally, physically and spiritually

Even though scientific research is still being done on the efficacy of essential oils to heal and cure people, especially when they are suffering from viral, fungal and bacterial infections, it has been proven through the millenniums that many of these essential oils have plenty of therapeutic benefits and potential.

Millenniums ago, Dioscorides when compiling his De Materia Medica spoke about distilled essential oils, to heal. Steam distillation was in vogue in the 11$^{th}$ century, in the East, from where the Crusaders brought back the knowledge how to extract essential oils from flowers, roots, seeds, and leaves back to Europe.

# How Are Essential Oils Used in Aromatherapy?

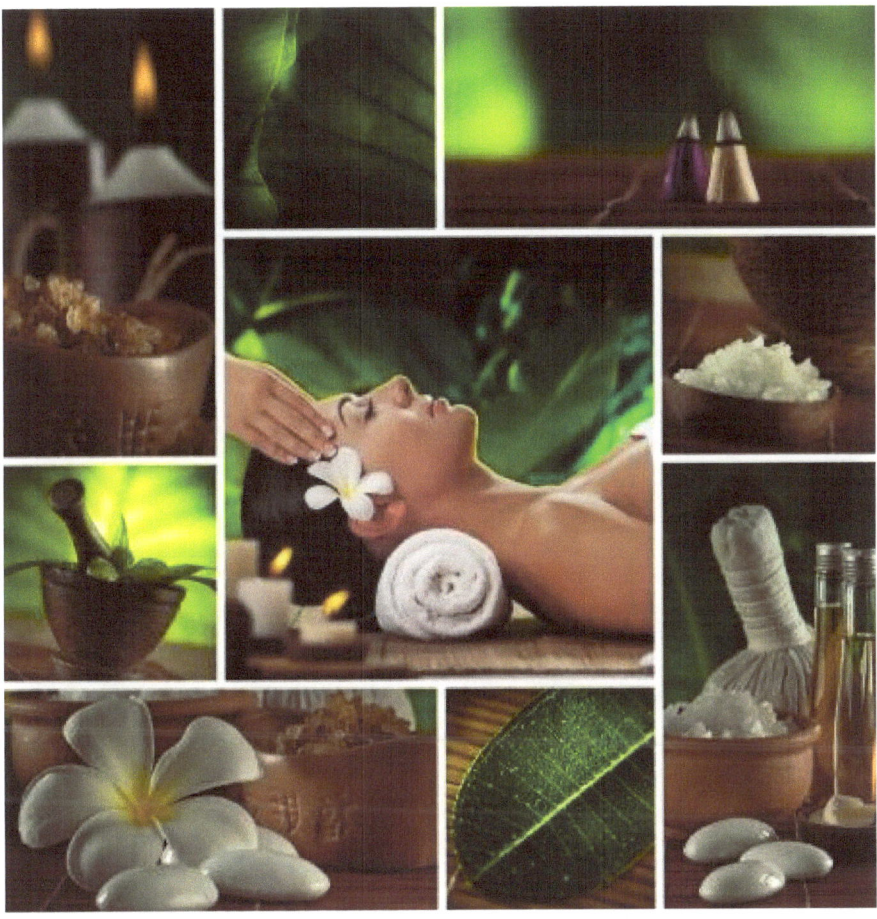

Essential oils are normally used with the help of a diffuser. Diffusion in the air, can be done by burning these essential oils, and allowing them to spread their fragrance to the atmosphere. Also, this fumigation is going to help in disinfection.

Direct inhalation of these oils is excellent for chest infection, and clearing up chronic conditions. Also, some of these essential oils are considered to be very effective in enhancing your mood, and causing you to relax. You can consider these to be the psychological effects of the sweet smelling oils.

Topical use of these essential oils is done in compresses, massage, skin care, and also in baths.

Aromatherapy does not cure chronic conditions. However, it helps heal the body, and strengthen the auto immune system. So a person may consider himself healed because of aromatherapy.

For example lemon oil is considered to be an excellent way to relieve stress, along with lavender oil. You may also want to inhale Rosemary oil, to relax yourself. Peppermint and Jasmine oil are excellent antidepressants.

In fact, I cannot resist inhaling Jasmine oil, just like as if I am inhaling sal volatile, every night, just for sheer fun. And because I like the aroma! Whether it relaxes me or not, I am not very certain, but I feel like I have been taken into an atmosphere of luxurious, sumptuous and opulent living! If it makes me feel happy, then why not?

Also, one drop of this essential oil or any of your other favorites added to your bath water is going to keep you sweetly scented, and fresh throughout the day.

# Best Oils for Your Skin

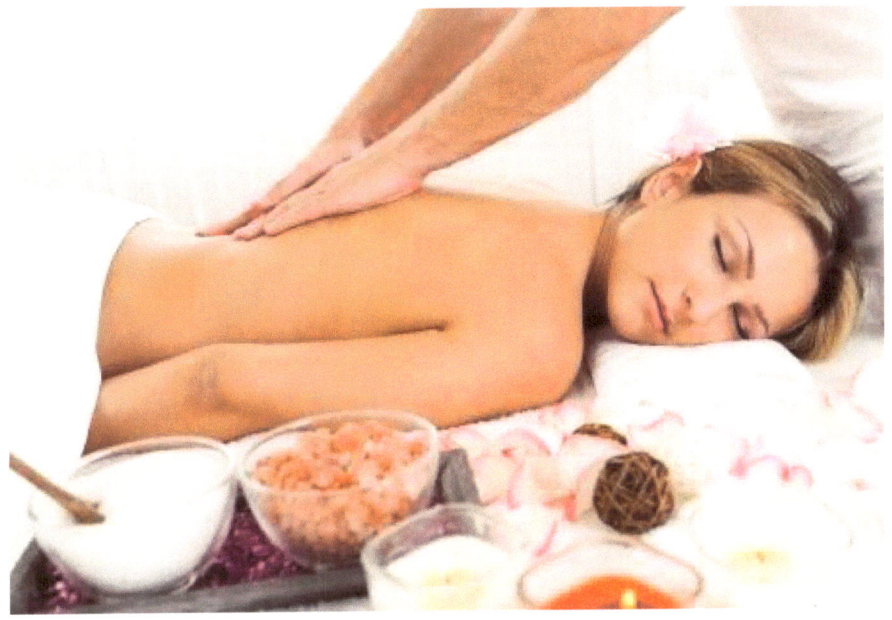

The best oils to use on your face and body are definitely ones which have excellent therapeutic qualities. Some of the best oil choices are almond oil, wheat germ oil and olive oil. These oils are rich in vitamins and are nourishing. Wheat germ oil is comparatively stronger smelling, because it is after all an extract from a grain. So use it in very small quantities.

If you do not mind stronger smelling oils, you can use coconut and mustard oil, especially for massaging your body. These oils are normally used in the East, to massage the limbs of the old, young and also babies. The idea is that this regular massage promotes muscular growth, and keeps the skin healthy and glowing and well-nourished. After that, the oil is allowed to permeate into the skin for about two hours before one takes a cold water bath.

If you are massaging this oil in the winter, remember to take a warm water bath; extremely hot water dries up the skin, and makes it flaky.

# Knowing More about Essential Oils

The list of natural essential oils obtained from flowers, petals, bark, seeds, leaves, and other parts of the plant are too numerous to be described here. However, you can see an extensive and very useful list here.

http://en.wikipedia.org/wiki/List_of_essential_oils

Here are some of the flowers from where you can derive volatile oils – lavender, jasmine, rose, rosemary, geraniums and carnations. The expensive rose essential oil that you buy in the market today is 90% geranium oil and 10% rose oil.

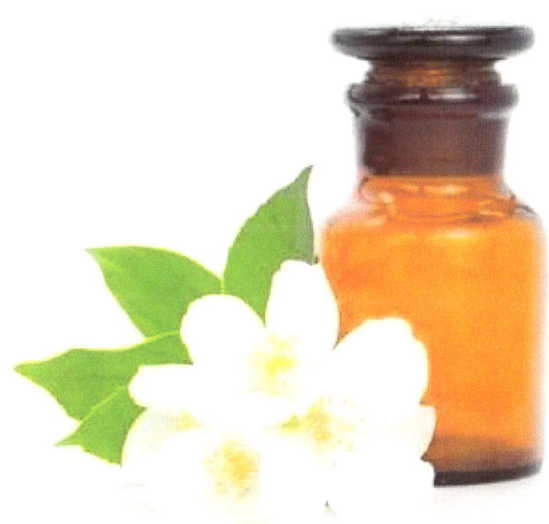

Plants from where you can get essential oils from the leaves and stem – basil family, lemongrass, geranium, cinnamon, patchouli and verbena.

Bark – Cassia, Eucalyptus and cinnamon.

Wood – Sandalwood pine, cedar.

Roots – Sassafras, valerian, Angelica

Seeds – coriander, nutmeg, fennel, caraway, aniseed and dill.

Fruits – lemon, orange, Juniper and bergamot.

Roots and rhizomes – ginger, orris, calamus.

Gums – myrrh and Peru balsam.

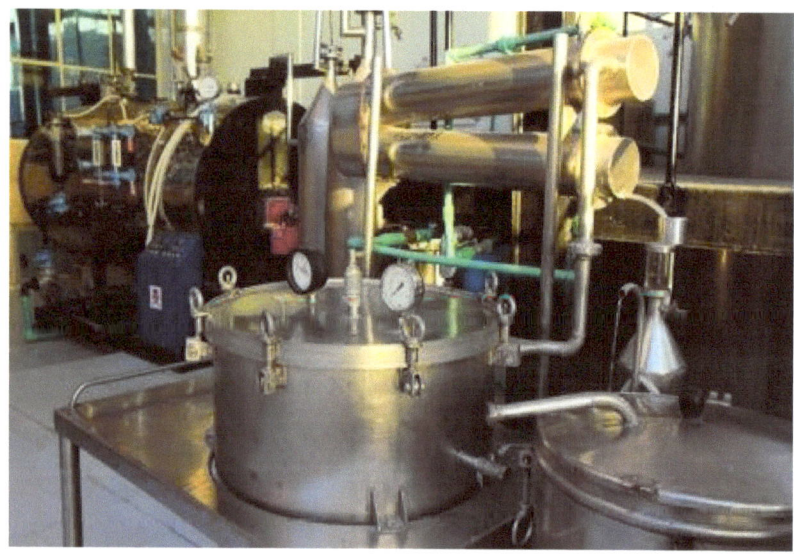

**Essential oil Distillation is a very complicated process**

# Where Are Essential Oils Used?

The sweet smelling soaps which you use, the perfumes which you spray, the confectioneries which you eat, alcoholic beverages, food products, detergents , and even pesticides use essential oils in some quantity or the other.

There was a time when it was very difficult to extract, essential oils from plants, especially when technological development was just limited to distillation. Steam distillation, water distillation and maceration are the ancient ways in which you can extract essential oils from plants.

Distillation works excellently for rose blossoms and rose petals. On the other hand, if you are faced with delicate flowers like Jasmine, Hyacinth and tuberose, the traditional extraction method is going to be solvent extraction. Sturdier volatile oils like citronella can be extracted with extremely good results through water distillation.

# Infused oils

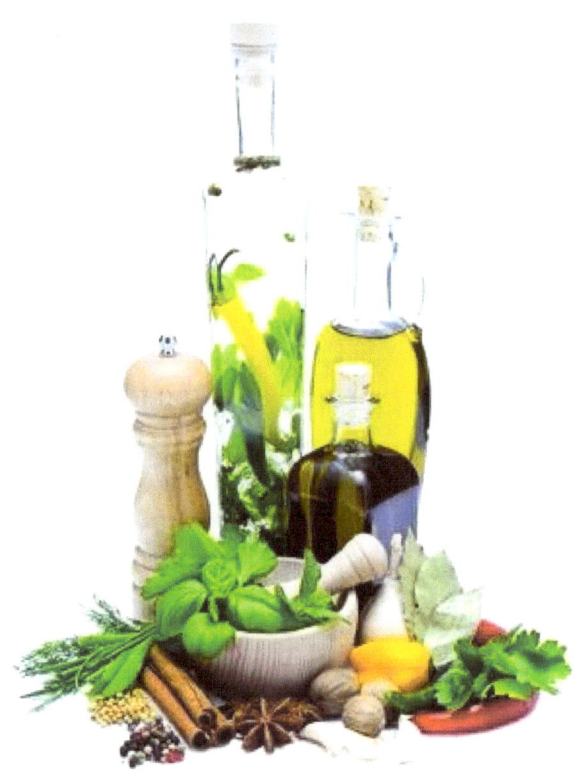

**Olive Oil Is Excellent As a Carrier Oil**

Somebody while talking about beauty products said that she made essential oils. Sorry, you cannot "make" essential oils, because they are natural. What she meant was that she was infusing oils with an oil base, and the essential oils taken from other plants, all mixed up together, in one mixture. This base mixture is then used to make other products, especially ointments, salves and a unguents. This base oil is called the carrier oil. Normally, you use a cooking oil, or another neutral oil like olive oil as a carrier oil, in which you are going to infuse the essential oils of flowers, spices and other volatile oil bearing parts of the plant.

Now there are two types of making infused oils, the sun method or the working lady method! The slow sun method is for that lady, who has a beautiful garden with lots of sunlight streaming in. The working lady method is, of course, for the lady who does not have time to breathe and as she is working on a tight time schedule, wants everything done like man, yesterday! *(You know, my sort of Worker Bee, always looking for shortcuts done everywhere, so this can be done best on a Sunday!)*

# The Slow Sun Method

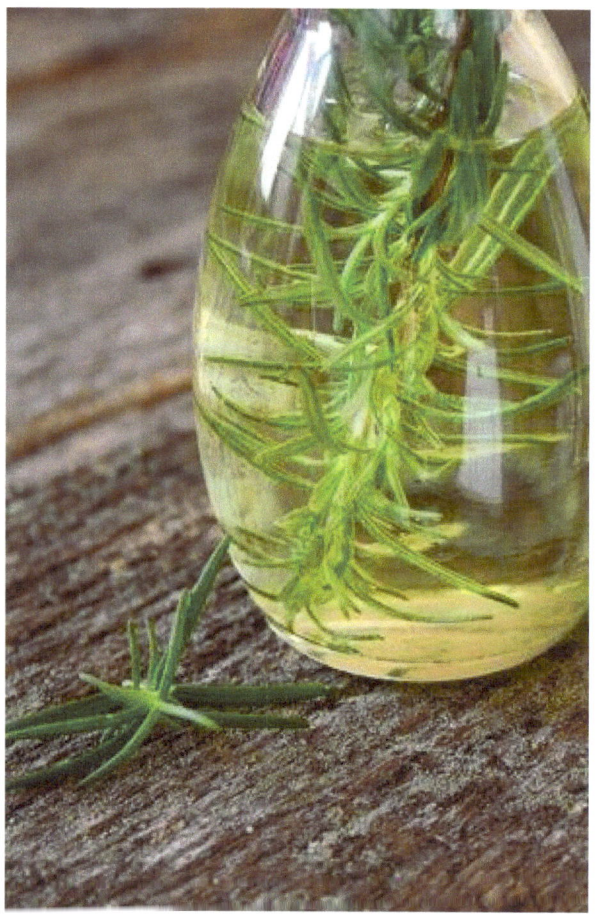

**Place this in the sun, here I am making an infusion of roses.**

I normally choose a light vegetable oil like sunflower oil, but my grandmother used to infuse herbs in desi ghee (Clarified butter) or freshly homemade butter like her grandmother used to do. Ancient wise women of the East and the West also used goose grease, and lard to make these infused oils.

I have noticed that the desi ghee infusions are more powerful, because of their concentrated power to heal. But then everybody knows my always to let pockets would screech blue murder if I spent lots of money on pure and expensive desi ghee, just for the sole purpose of using it in infusions instead of eating it and so gaining full value for my money , so if you do have a good supply of homemade desi ghee , be my guest and use it !

By the way somehow, everybody in the many parts of the Indian subcontinent knows that desi ghee is the best agent for painless healing of cuts and wounds.

*[How to make pure clarified butter- desi ghee? See the traditional manner in the Appendix.]*

Anyway, collect your flower petals -- red roses please- the ones which are so popular in making garlands and bouquets. Then, fill a large glass jar ( we call it a pickle jar bottle) with a good vegetable oil, or homemade butter or ghee.

Add the rose petals until they are covered with the oil but are not tightly packed, (I found out that three -- 4 handfuls of the petals did me just fine, there was enough of space for all of them to breathe.)

Cover with an air tight lid and leave in direct sunshine. The rose petals will turn brown after a couple of days. Remove them and add fresh blooms. Repeat this procedure until the oil is tinged pink. (The more changes you do, the more rose extract you are going to have in the oil in your precious bottle.)

People in sunny areas of the world are very lucky because they have a good supply of rose flowers as well as direct sunlight. But in most of the Western countries, it is tough luck when all ye  sun deprived  people have to go up to 20 or more changes because of the uncertain summer season and rainy weather.  The more you persevere, and the more patient you are, the more this rather long method captures the fragrance of the delicate flower.

## Quick Kitchen Method

## Rosewater through Steam Condensation

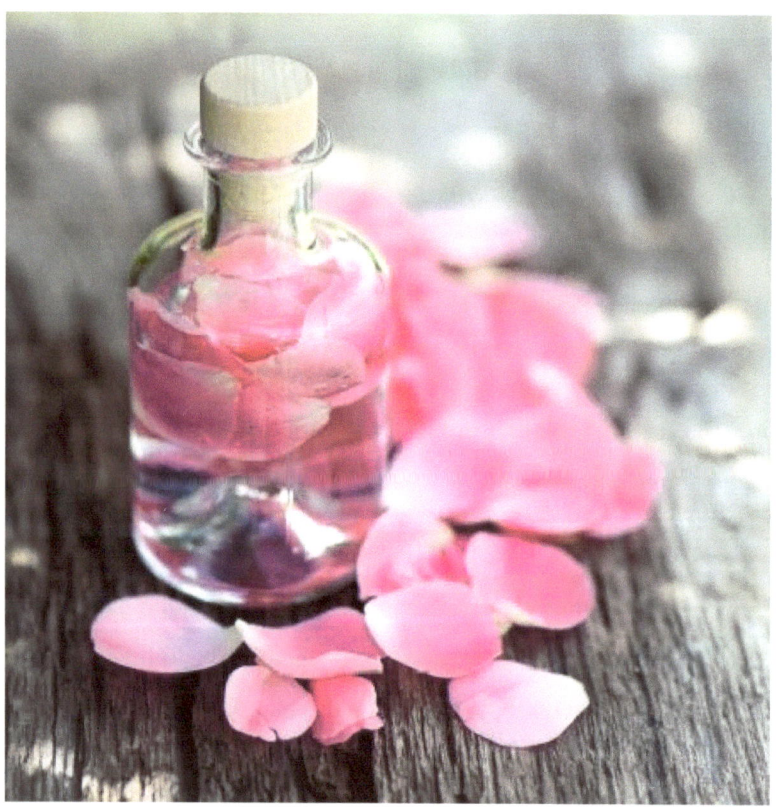

This is the process, with which people in the East have been making **gulab-jal (rose water)** and also to extract essential oils from herbs

The essential oil is going to float on the surface of the condensed water. It is going to be into minute a quantity, so you can have those perfumed droplets float over the surface of your bottle of fresh homemade rosewater.

**For this method, you need to have a large supply of rose petals , and lots of ice handy!**

Take a large cooking  pot, insert a clean brick or rock in its bottom , fill  the pot with rose petals ,-the more the merrier,- or  herbs around the brick. Cover with water and place a small glass dish on top of the brick.

Put a stainless steel bowl on top of the pot and fill with ice. Simmer about three hours depending how many petals or herbs you have, replacing the ice as needed. The bowl with the ice will condense the steam which will then drip down into the glass bowl. The water in the glass bowl is your rose water -or whatever herb extract-, and on top  will be a pure layer of oil. This is the essential oil. You can separate these and use the water in cooking, or as Gulab jal  and the essential oil in lotions, soaps or whatever.

And this is the precious extract, which is sold in the market for 50 $  every 10g!

This rosewater is one of the most essential commodities of every self-respecting young Eastern and Oriental beauty's arsenal.  Not only does this moisturize  the skin and keep it silky and soft, but it also imparts a soft scented fragrance, which is more appealing than the heavy musky and expensive perfumes, which are alas, so often a regular and cloying substitute for neglected ablutions.

# Method Two – Heating Method

For this, you will have to have all the petals as well as a vegetable oil ready.

**1 1/2 cups of vegetable oil and 250 grams of petals gave me 1 1/2 cups of infused oil.**

•Place half of the rose petals and all the oil in a container with a tight lid.

•Put a container in a pan, fill the pan up with water to within 1 inch of the top of the container and simmer this slowly for 2 hours. This water bath makes sure that your precious oil is exposed to prolonged heating without spoiling the oil by burning or boiling. To save time and energy costs, I normally boil 2-3 airtight containers together.

•After two hours, allow the mixture to cool slightly and then strain it well. Now, we are just halfway through the process and the infusion has changed color.

At this strength, this infusion is mild enough to use as baby oil or bath oil. Refill the canister with the remaining rose petals, cover with the strained oil and return to the water bath. Simmer gently for another two hours. Don't forget to replace the lid! Also make sure to check the water level to make sure that the water has not boiled away completely. Nobody has any use for burnt oil.

When the oil has cooked enough, pour it through a muslin cloth or very fine strainer. If you are using fresh petals, there might be some watery liquid at the bottom of the oil. Remember to separate out this liquid and throw it away, because it is quite certain to spoil the oil if it is left unattended.

Once the oil has been strained , gather all the petals in the cloth and wring them out to extract every drop of oil . This oil will keep fresh for a year but it will eventually become rancid. Many cosmetologists thus add some wheat germ oil to delay the spoiling process -- (about 25 g.)

As for the spent petals, I do not throw them away, but I put them into my bathwater so as not to waste them! These oils have to be poured into clean bottles. Remember to store them away in dark and not transparent bottles in a cool and dark place away from the sunlight.

I normally make marigold, rose and cayenne infusions at one go, thus saving lots of time, energy and fuel.

# Making Salves from Essential Infused Oils

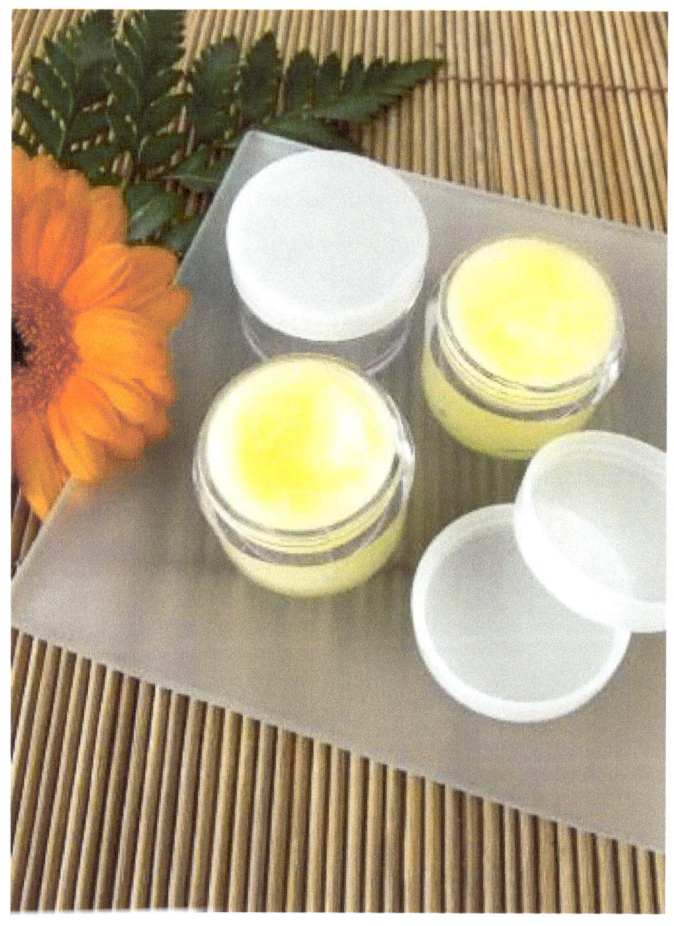

Now, that you have already infused oils, you would like to make some natural salves from them.

A salve is the oil thickened with beeswax, melted together in the ratio of 4:1 .

Use the same hot water heating system of one utensil in another to heat the beeswax and the oil together so that they do not get burnt in direct heat.

Rose and Marigold salves are excellent to make your skin smoother. Damaged and inflamed skin can also be healed by these salves. I use rose salve in the summer and Marigold in the winter or whenever I hurt myself. Forget about Savlon or Dettol for these mild cuts and bruises.

Solid salves can be made for damaged, chapped and even inflamed skin, as well as for treating hemorrhoids, by thickening the oil mixture into a salve with beeswax in a 4 to 1 ratio. Try making a rose salve for your lips in the winter and a Marigold salve for cuts, burns, and scratches.

## Marigold Healing Salve

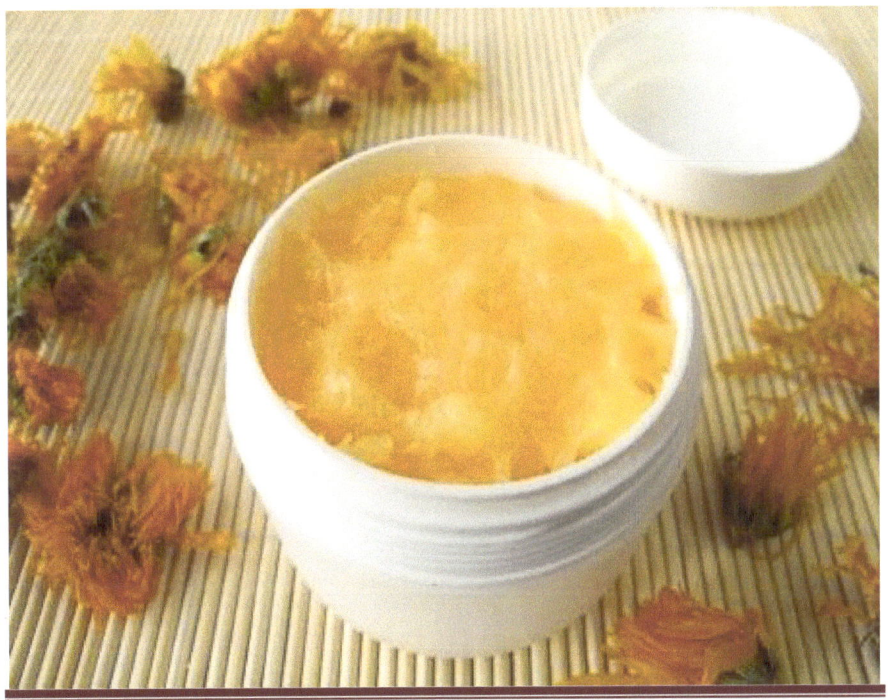

I once made a paste of marigolds, and put them up on a cut. It was very soothing and healed it well. And then I used a paste of turmeric and Marigold to remove the scar. This ointment can easily be made at home by washing marigolds well and pounding them freshly with turmeric to make a paste. Then boil them in one cup of oil, for about two hours. You have a healing oil, which can then be applied to the mild cuts and bruises and then bandaged up. But as I am making it into a salve, I am going to add 40 g of that oil to 10 g of beeswax. Heat over water, so that the wax is melted and mixed up thoroughly with the oil. Place in a glass bottle, and apply whenever you suffer from cuts, bruises, and wounds, which you do not want scarred.

Traditional salves were normally made with butter, bear's fat, and goose grease. But as we are much more civilized, we use other carriers like strained vegetable shortening. These herbs are infused into the fats in the same way as they are infused into the oils.

When the fats cooled down, they naturally became a solid and beneficial cream.

# Chest Oil

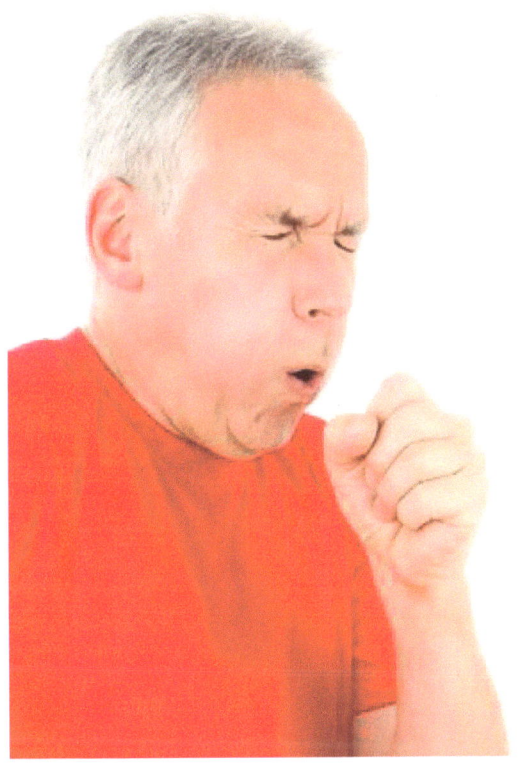

This is a traditional remedy, which you are going to use when you are suffering from infected, dry coughs. As I do not have bears grease, I am going to be using 11/4 cups of vegetable oil. This is excellent for asthmatic patients, especially children. Rub it all over the back, front and chest of the affected patient, especially between the shoulder blades, before the child goes to sleep.

Take 1/4 ounces – about 1 teaspoon – each of aniseed lavender and thyme. Now add three cloves of crushed garlic for adults, and one sliced onion for children. Add a pinch of ground ginger.

Powder, and mix all these ingredients together and make into an infused oil. Use this as soon as people suffering from chest infections begin showing the symptoms. This is going to heal the infection and prevent it from spreading or getting aggravated.

# What Is the Difference between a Salve and an Ointment

Salves are normally made up of infused oils and beeswax. Ointments have only fats and oils, thickened with wax. The ratios are different. You are going to put 10 quantities of oil to one quantity of wax to make up an ointment. The ratio for a salve is 4:1 with four quantities of oil, to one quantity of wax.

You can use any wax to make of these salves and ointments, as long as they are pure. Paraffin wax and even candle wax have been known to be used in the making of ointments. However, serious herbalists use only beeswax, as it brings extra natural healing properties during the preparation of the product.

# Simple Perfumed Ointments

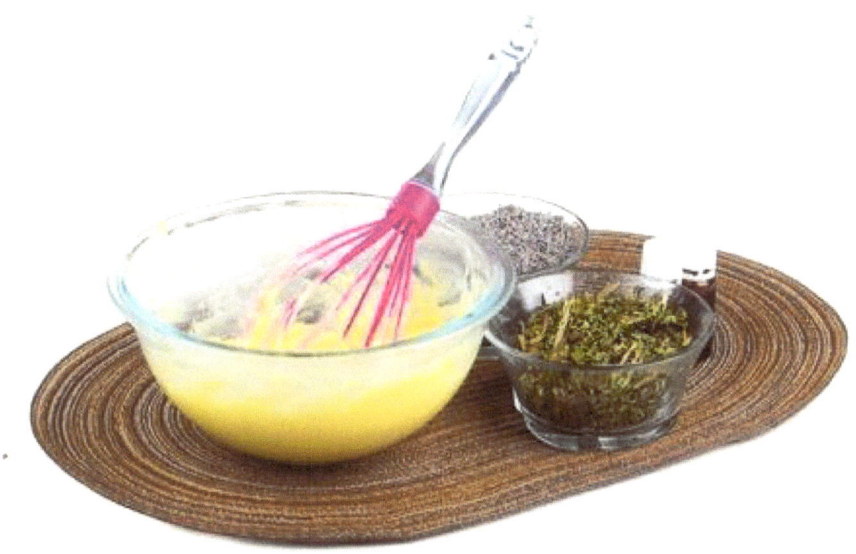

A couple of days ago, I prepared my month's quota of face cream ointment by melting one part of beeswax in 10 parts of Rose infused oil , in a container which was put into a bath.

 I was astonished when it took only 10 minutes for the beeswax to melt, after continuous stirring to make sure that it did not get burned. After all, I had spent four hours, in extracting that infused oil from those rose petals. I put the ointment into a glass jar. Plastic jars are a complete no-no for natural products.

Take out your handy container and place the infused oil and beeswax cut into small pieces in the ratio of 10:1. [250 g oil:25 g beeswax] Stand the container in the larger water pan. Carefully pour water into the larger water pan. Here you have to be careful that the level of the water is lower than that of the level of the oil, because this oil container is not going to have a lid upon it. Bring the water down to a gentle boil and then turn the heat down. On this slow simmering, the beeswax is melted by stirring it carefully with a metal spoon .

This ointment is removed and poured into clean jars before it starts to set. Do not fill it up to the brim. To make a smooth surface, wait till the whole of the ointment has solidified, melt some left over ointment in the water bath and top it up upon the solidified surface to make a smooth covering upon the brim.

This is such an easy way to make stylish perfumed ointments for the people you care, as gifts.

# Neem Oil and Ointment

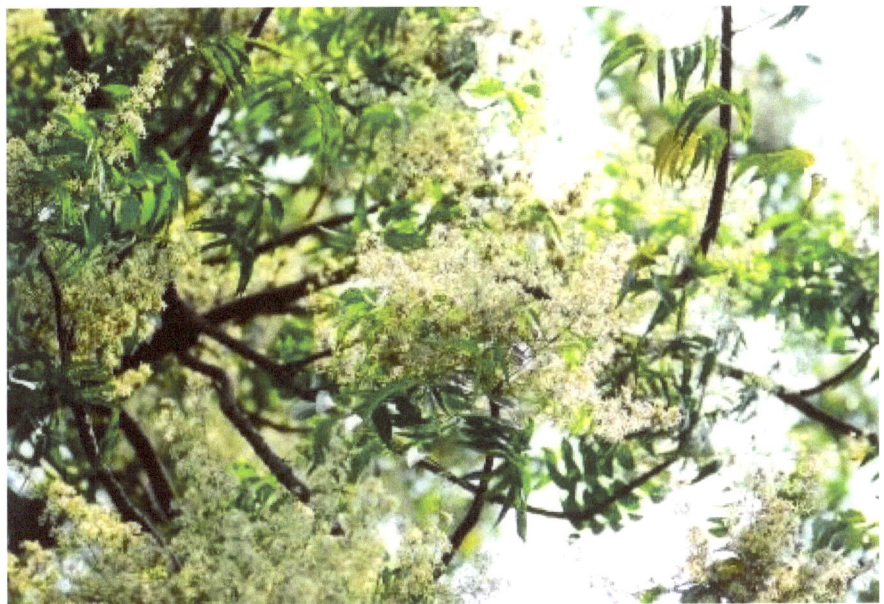

**Neem Oil is extracted from the neem tree**

Take three fistfuls of fresh green neem leaves and add them to 250 g of boiling hot oil. Allow to cook until all the leaves are burnt. Now this very powerful oil needs to be filtered, and placed in a glass bottle. This is an excellent remedy to apply on Burns and wounds, if you do not want to turn it into an ointment.

Here is my Neem ointment.

- **2/3 cups cooking oil,**
- **15 g beeswax, grated or chopped into small pieces,**
- **50 g infused oil (25 grams for Neem)**

Put the oils, and beeswax in the into a small pan. Put the lid on and stand it into the large water pan . Carefully pour water into the larger water pan. Here you have to be careful that the level of the water is lower than that of the level of the oil, because this oil container is not going to have a lid upon it. Keep stirring until the wax is melted.

Allow to cool a little, take out the inner pan and remove the lid. Put this ointment in a handy container and use it to heal wounds. Naturally, these ointments keep for many months.

You may ask me if I have tried making ointments out of Neem oil, so plentiful in the East. The answer is yes, and it works equally well. But I use only about 25 g of Neem oil, because it is very powerful and very concentrated.

# Healing Ointment

The ointment recipe I gave to you above is for wound infection prevention, but this is an effective remedy to prevent burns from getting infected .

**Add 250 g of Neem oil to 125 g of wax. Now add 1 kg of fresh green Neem leaves juice, 50 g of powdered Neem root bark and 25 g of dried Neem leaf ash.** I do not think I have left anything out in this very powerful concoction!

Now, heat the oil with the liquid on slow heat until the oil is reduced to half its quantity. Now add the wax. Then both of them have turned into us. Most mixture, you are going to add the Neem root powder and the ash.

Just heat for another one minute and cool. This is the best remedy in which you can cure bun infections. Try it out right now.

In fact, I have this in my kitchen, because that is the place where I get burnt ever so often through oil splats and by accidentally touching red-hot utensils.

Also, when the burns are healed, I get rid of the scars, by a mixture of turmeric paste with honey.

# Liniments

In the winter, I made a cayenne liniment ( 10 tsps full of red cayenne pepper oil. Add a mixture of alcohol and water in a  1:1 ratio) for rubbing the joints in hot – arthritic conditions.  Now, this milder liniment is more useful, because imagine pouring concentrated infusions of red pepper upon a delicate skin. Thanks to this liniment, the oldies of the family breeze through the winters without any joint pain.

Remember to shake the liniment bottle  well  before applying.

Let me just give you another trade secret of the pain balms used for aches and pains.  It is a mixture of ginger and cayenne put in a liniment of Rosemary infused  oil!

Cayenne infused oils, along with ginger is excellent for winter massaging, especially on painful joints. You would want to add a little bit of powdered cinnamon to this infusion, while preparing the oil.

Remember that the oils that use for making herbal infusions should be light and odorless. This is so that they do not drown out the natural fragrance and aroma of the herbs, spices and volatile oils.

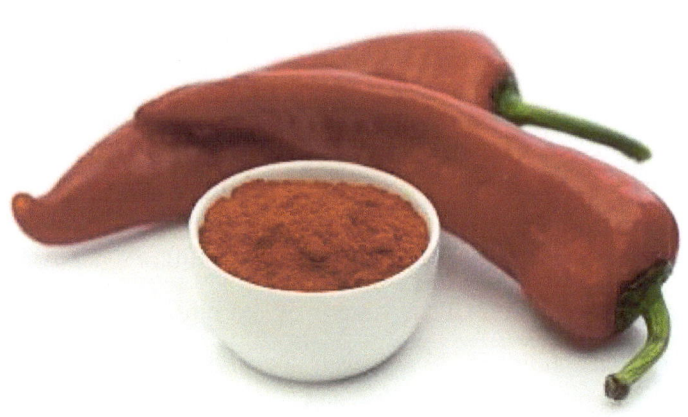

## Tips and Precautions about Essential Oils

Remembered that essential oils are highly concentrated. So even a few drops of essential oil in a pure and unadulterated form can cause harm when it comes in contact with your skin. That is why essential oils are always diluted before they are used.

If you are using essential oils for topical applications, you can use coconut oil, olive oil, as well as jojoba.

Using essential oils over a long period of time in one particular spot can cause skin damage. That is because of allergies, especially due to the use of chemical pesticides, thanks to inorganic methods used in farming in the 21$^{st}$ century.

Many essential oils are highly toxic, so make sure that you do not ingest them. Evening Primrose oil, however, can be taken internally, to help heal dry skin conditions. Also, the essential oils found in vegetable oils, and in leafy vegetables are definitely not harmful, because they are rich source of vitamins and essential minerals and nutrients.

Essential oils should not be taken by expectant mothers or mothers who are nursing. Sunflower, safflower, peanut and grape seed oils are fixed and essential oils, which are extremely healthy. They are colorless, light, and odorless, so they can be used as excellent carriers. So use them when you are making infused oils.

Do not ever take eucalyptus, Sage, cedar or hyssop essential oils internally. Accidents normally happen when these oils are left unattended in the presence of children. Also, there are some essential oils like Wintergreen , which react adversely, when interacting with normal drugs. So if you are taking anticoagulants, ask your doctor if you can apply Wintergreen topically or internally.

# Appendix

## How to make  Desi Ghee

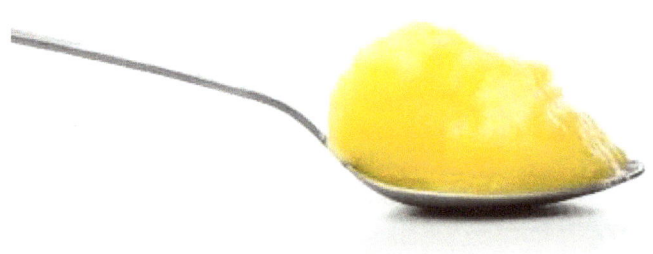

As more and more scientific researchers in the West are proving that clarified butter is the best healing ingredient found in nature, is it surprising that the ancients of yore used this very powerful concentrated butter as a carrier base, especially to heal and to make beauty products? Any land of milk and honey would have very healthy people, because they would have been brought up on a diet of plenty of fresh milk, butter, butter, yogurt, cheese, milk and clarified butter.

Start collecting cream from your daily milk supply. 6 to 8 days, will give you enough of cream to make Desi ghee. Heat the milk cream, and you are going to find it melting into Desi ghee. The leftover sediment is delicious, when spread on Indian breads, Pita breads, or over any spicy dish.

Villagers traditionally make Desi ghee in Asia by adding yogurt to the cream for a week or so. They intend to turn it into buttermilk, fresh butter and Desi ghee by churning. This turning process has three stages. Add water to the yoghurt cream mixture and you get buttermilk and butter. Heat the butter and you are going to get Desi ghee.

Remember to remove the sediment from the top, when you store this Desi ghee in airtight glass bottles. The sediment is delicious on breads with honey. One tablespoonful of this highly concentrated powerful oil spread on every meal surface, including vegetables, pulses and beans – every available visible surface – and eaten every day is considered to be the reason why so many people stay healthy in the villages of Asia. This is, of course, supported with plenty of hard physical work throughout the day.

# Conclusion

The magic of essential oils has given you a lot of information about the use of essential oils in healing, and in keeping you beautiful. Many scientists still consider aromatherapy to be "quack" alternative medicine, because there is no scientific proof that people can be healed by inhaling fumes or getting themselves massaged with essential oils. Nevertheless, these essential oils have been in use to bring peace of mind, relaxation, and harmony in body and mind down the centuries. So one goes by what one feels, especially when one is inhaling something relaxing and sweet.

Also, essential oils in your healing salves and healing ointments are extremely good to keep you beautiful and healthy.

# Author Bio

**Dueep Jyot Singh** is a Management and IT Professional who managed to gather Postgraduate qualifications in Management and English and Degrees in Science, French and Education while pursuing different enjoyable career options like being an hospital administrator, IT,SEO and HRD Database Manager/ trainer, movie scriptwriter, theatre artiste and public speaker, lecturer in French, Marketing and Advertising, ex-Editor of Hearts On Fire (now known as Solstice) Books Missouri USA, advice columnist and cartoonist, publisher and Aviation School trainer, ex- moderator on Medico.in, banker, student councilor ,travelogue writer … among other things! One fine morning, she decided that she had enough of killing herself by Degrees and went back to her first love -- writing. It's more enjoyable! She already has 48 published academic and 14 fiction- in- different- genre books under her belt.

When she is not designing websites or making Graphic design illustrations for clients , she is browsing through old bookshops hunting for treasures, of which she has an enviable collection – including R.L. Stevenson, O.Henry, Dornford Yates, Maurice Walsh, C.N.Williamson, Sapper, Bartimeus and the crown of her collection- Dickens "The Old Curiosity Shop," and so on… Just call her "Renaissance Woman" - collecting herbal remedies, acting like Universal Helping Hand/Agony Aunt, or escaping to her dear mountains for a bit of exploring, collecting herbs and plants, and trekking.

# Check out some of the other JD-Biz Publishing books

## Health Learning Series

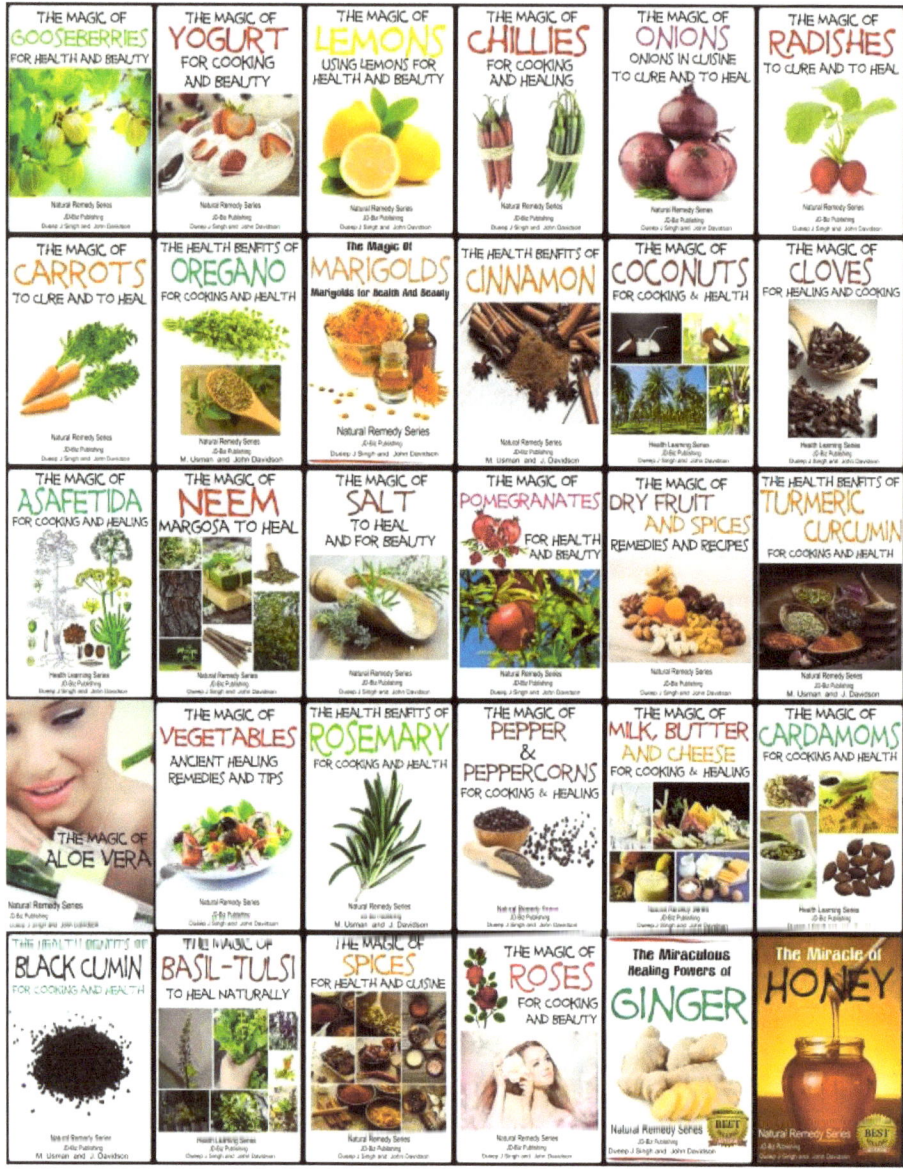

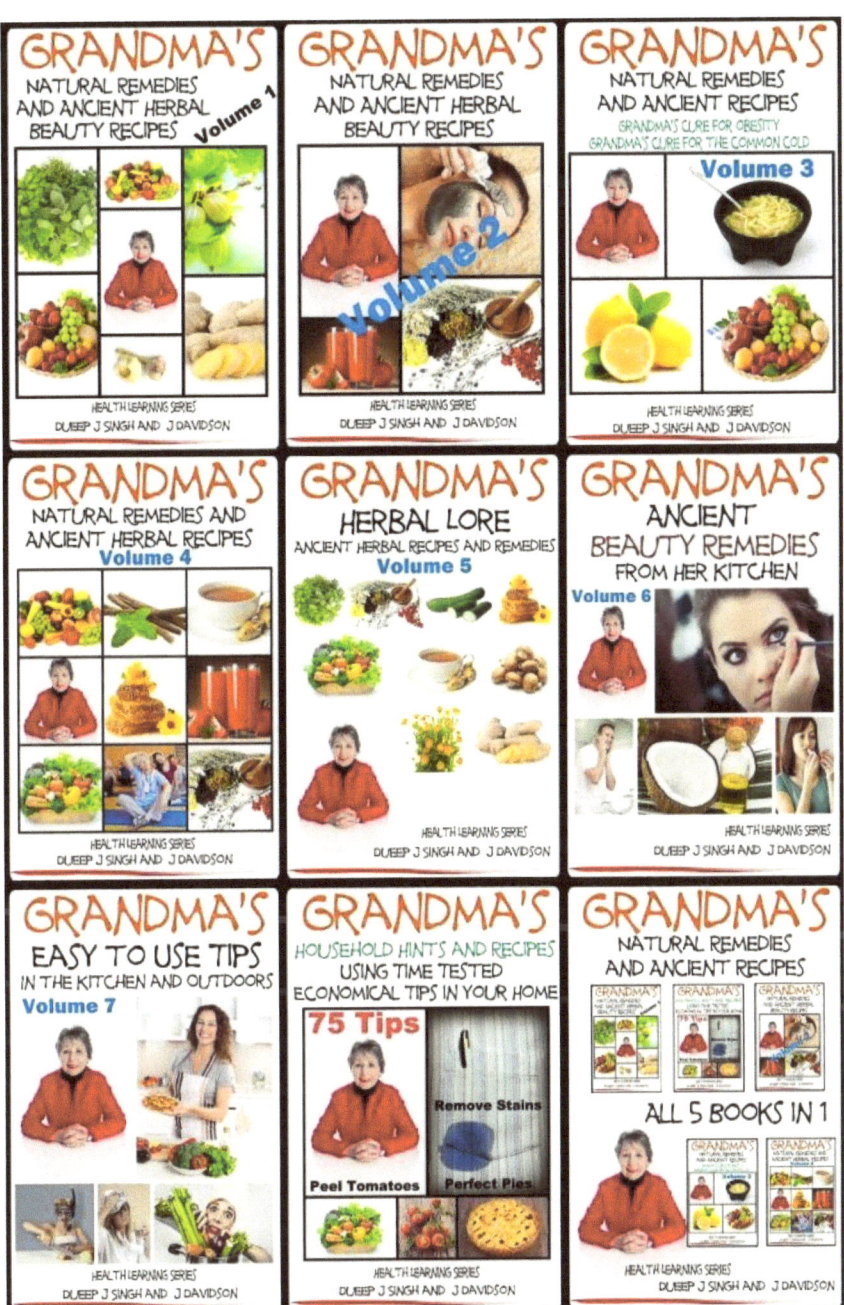

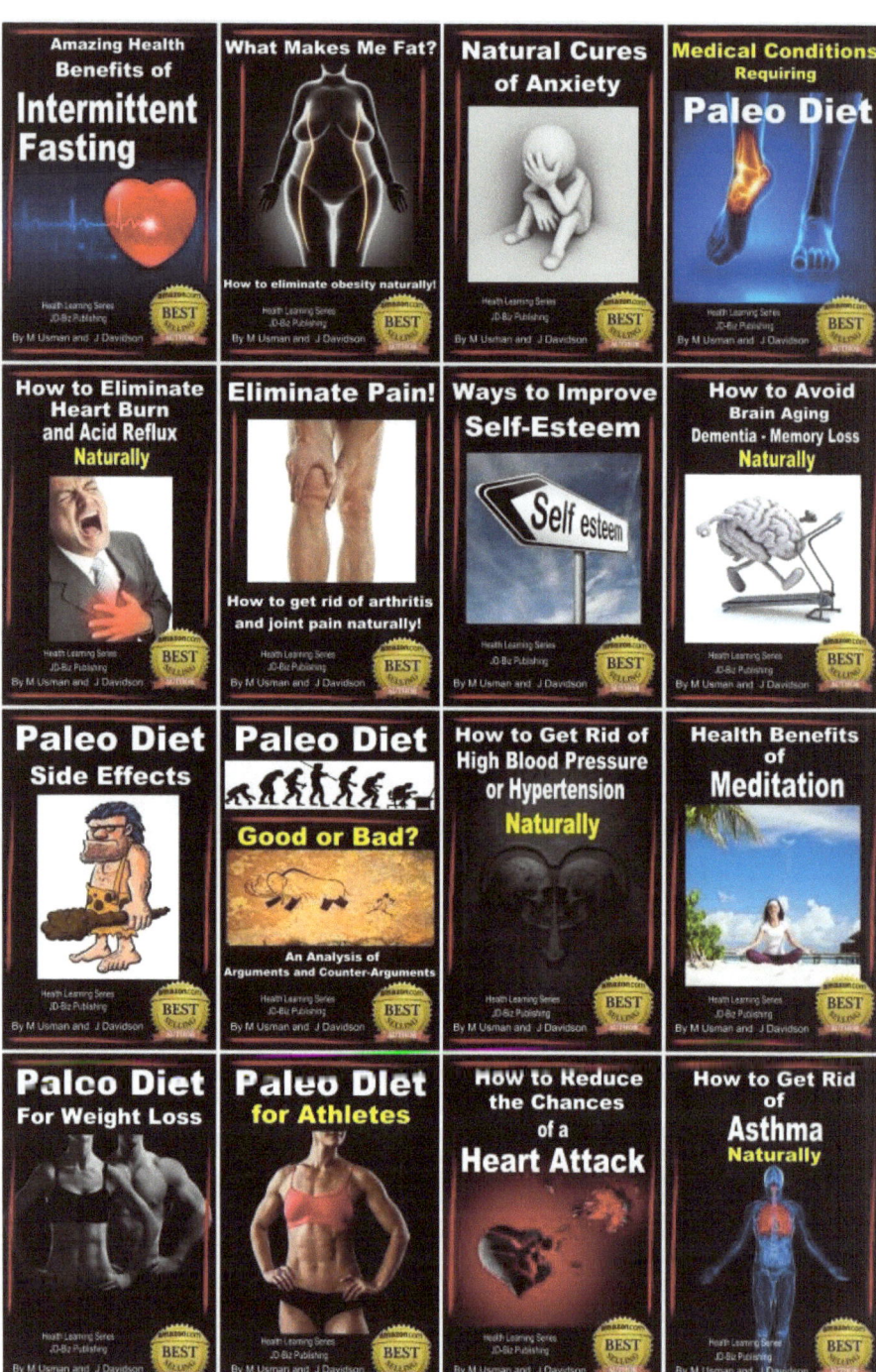

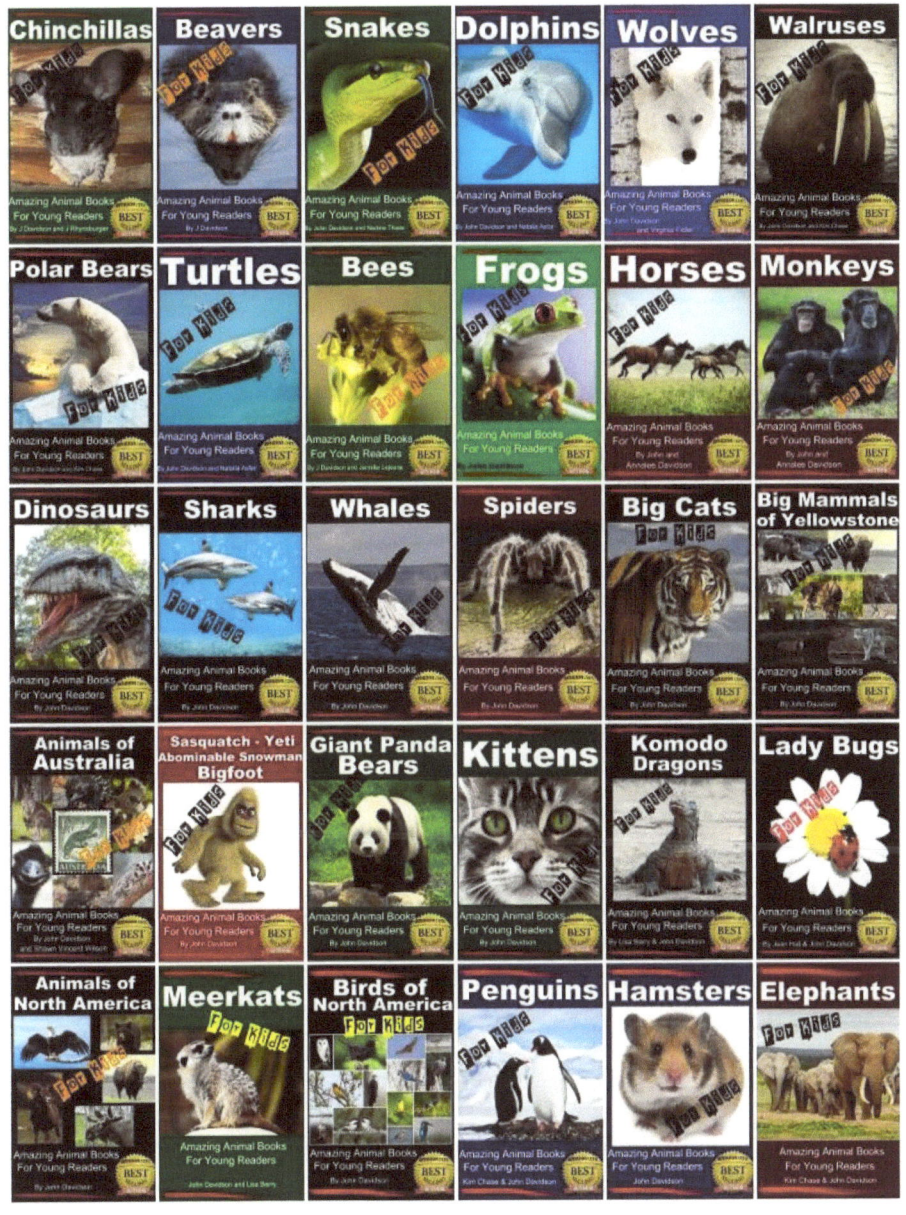

# Learn To Draw Series

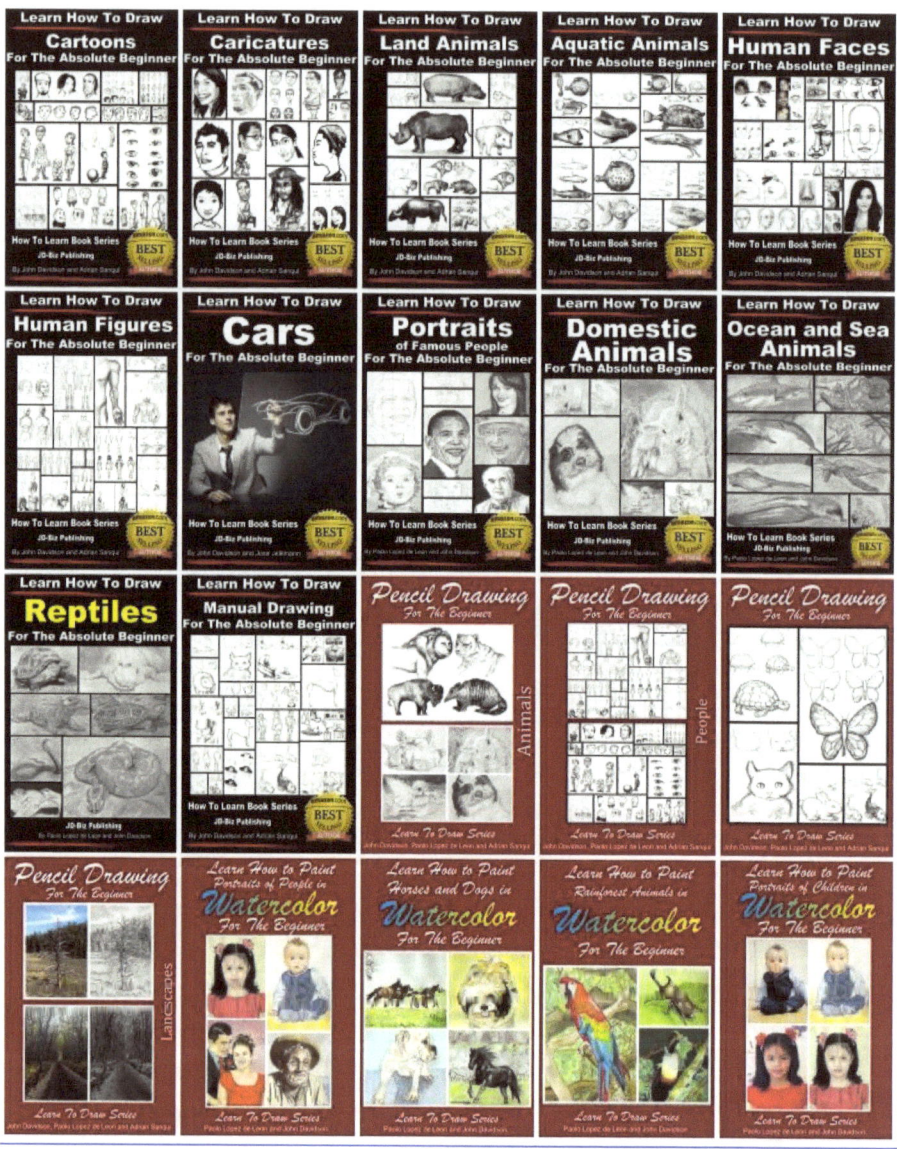

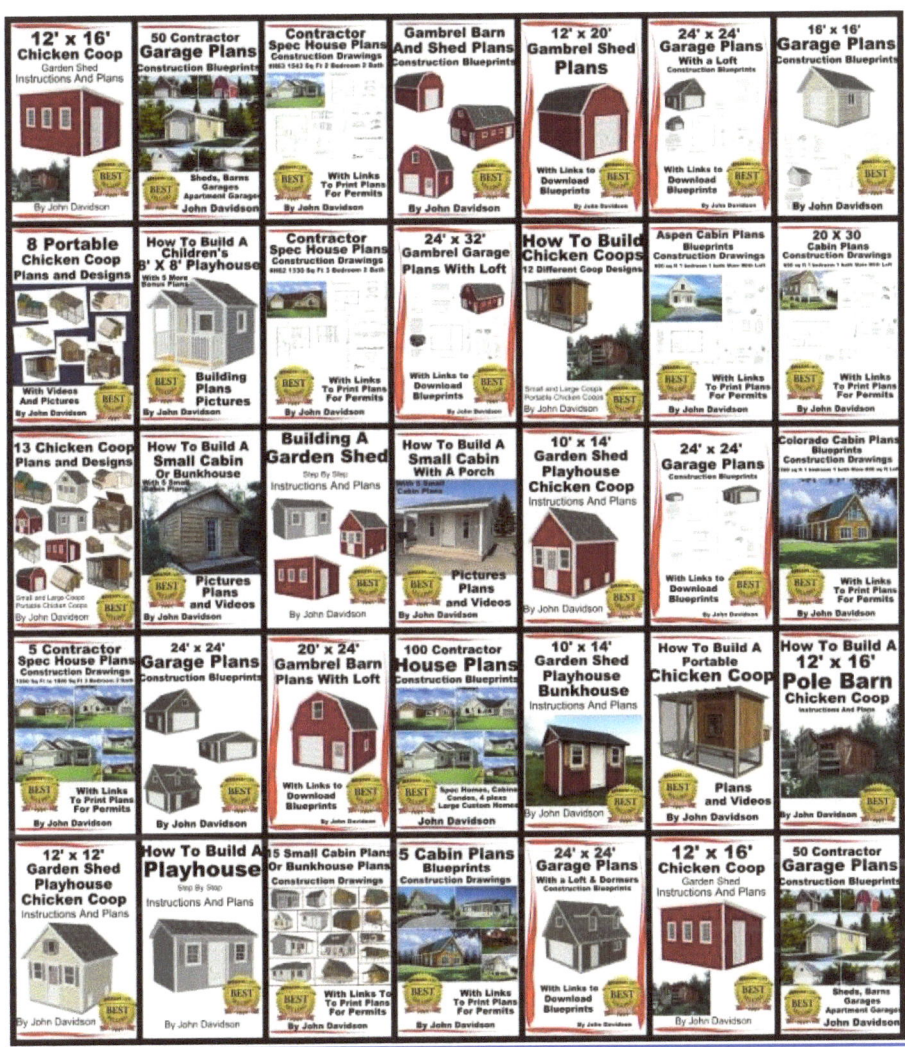

# Entrepreneur Book Series

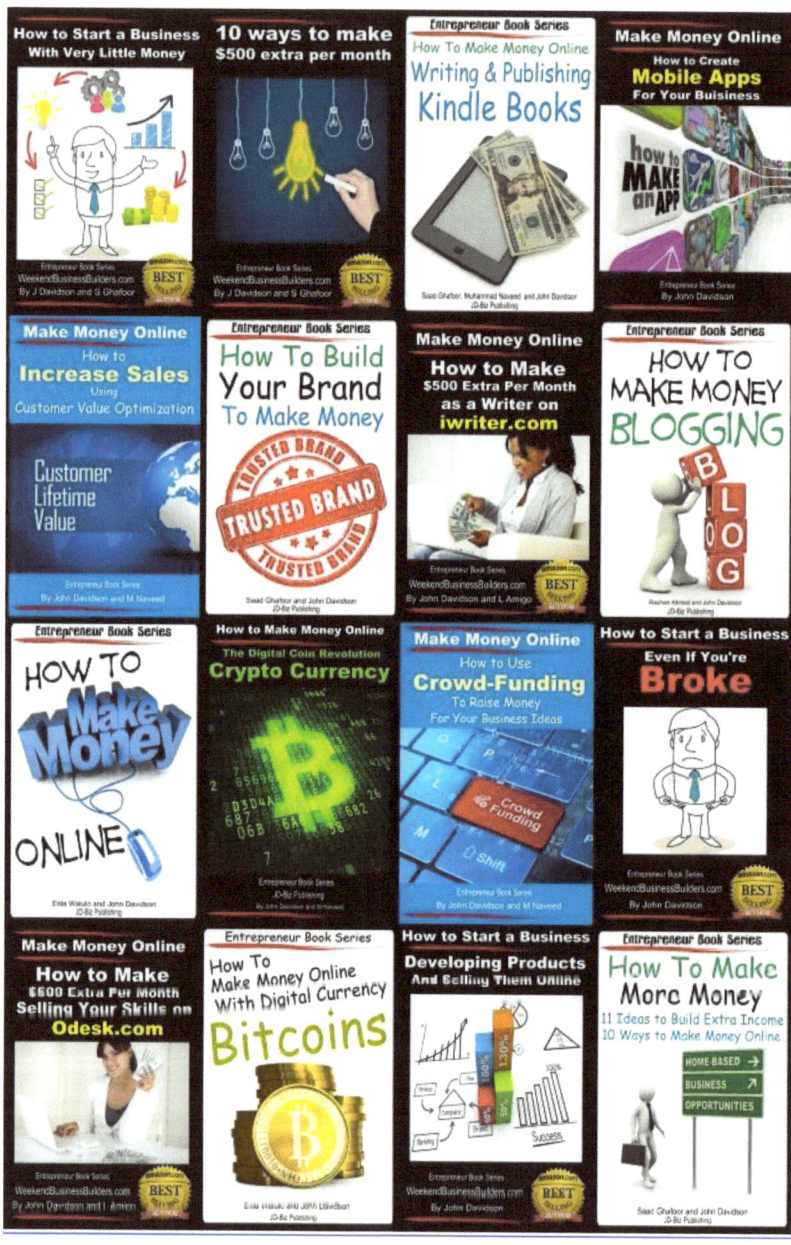

**Our books are available at**

1. Amazon.com

2. Barnes and Noble

3. Itunes

4. Kobo

5. Smashwords

6. Google Play Books

# Download Free Books!

# http://MendonCottageBooks.com

# Publisher

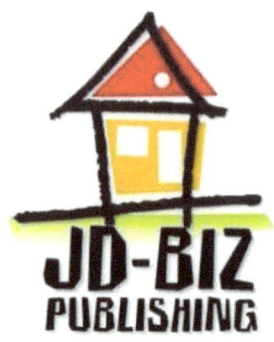

JD-Biz Corp

P O Box 374

Mendon, Utah 84325

http://www.jd-biz.com/

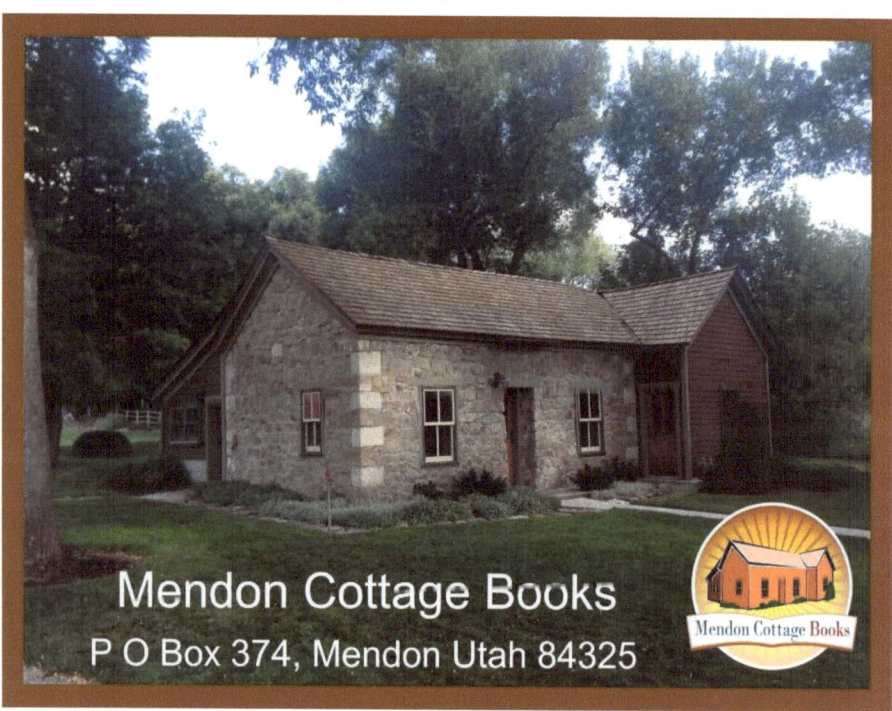

www.ingramcontent.com/pod-product-compliance
Lightning Source LLC
Chambersburg PA
CBHW050834290526
45792CB00001B/383